The Act Of Mastering Stress The Ultimate Guide to Overcoming Anxiety and Achieving.

Jessica Hensley

Table of contents

Chapter 1

What is stress and how it affects us

Stress is a natural and normal response to a perceived threat or challenge, whether it be physical or psychological. It's the body's way of mobilizing its resources to deal with a perceived threat or danger. In small doses, stress can be helpful and can actually improve our performance and focus. However, when stress becomes chronic or overwhelming, it can have a negative impact on our health and well-being.

When we experience stress, our body releases hormones such as cortisol and adrenaline, which trigger a range of physical responses including increased heart rate, rapid breathing, and muscle tension. These responses are part of the "fight or flight" response that prepares our body to either confront the perceived threat or run away from it.

However, when stress becomes chronic or prolonged, these physical responses can cause wear and tear on our body and contribute to a range of health problems. Chronic stress has been linked to an increased risk of heart disease, stroke, diabetes, and other chronic health conditions. It can also have a negative impact on our mental health, leading to symptoms of anxiety, depression, and burnout.

In addition to the physical and mental health effects, stress can also impact our relationships, work performance, and overall quality of life. Therefore, it's important to learn effective strategies for managing stress and preventing it from becoming chronic or overwhelming.

Ways stress affects the body.

Stress affects the body in a variety of ways. When we experience stress, our body releases hormones such as cortisol and adrenaline, which trigger the "fight or flight" response. This response prepares the body to deal with a perceived threat or danger, but it can also have negative effects on our physical health when it is prolonged or chronic. Here are some of the ways stress can affect the body:

1. Increased heart rate and blood pressure: During the stress response, the heart rate and blood pressure increase, which can put a strain on the cardiovascular system over time.

2. Muscle tension: Stress can cause muscle tension and stiffness, which can contribute to headaches, back pain, and other physical discomfort.

3. Digestive problems: Stress can affect the digestive system, causing symptoms such as stomach pain, bloating, constipation, or diarrhea.

4. Weakened immune system: Chronic stress can weaken the immune system, making us more susceptible to illness and infection.

5. Sleep problems: Stress can interfere with sleep, making it difficult to fall asleep or stay asleep. Over time, chronic sleep deprivation can have negative effects on both physical and mental health.

6. Mental health problems: Chronic stress has been linked to an increased risk of anxiety, depression, and other mental health problems.

7. Reproductive problems: Stress can affect reproductive health in both men and women, potentially leading to fertility problems or sexual dysfunction.

These are just a few examples of how stress can affect the body. By learning effective strategies for managing stress, we can help prevent these negative effects and maintain our physical and mental health.

Chapter 2

Common causes of stress in daily life. Tips for improving sleep hygiene to reduce stress.

Sure, I'd be happy to help with that. Here are some common causes of stress in daily life:

1. Work-related stress: The demands and pressures of work can often cause stress, whether it's from deadlines, heavy workloads, difficult colleagues or bosses, or long hours.

2. Financial stress: Financial worries, such as debt, job loss, or unexpected expenses, can be a significant source of stress for many people.

3. Relationship stress: Problems with family, friends, or romantic partners can cause significant stress, whether it's due to conflicts, breakups, or other issues.

4. Health-related stress: Illness, injury, or chronic health conditions can cause stress, as can concerns about health or the health of loved ones.

5. Time-related stress: Feeling like there's not enough time in the day to accomplish everything that needs to be done can be a source of stress for many people.

6. Major life changes: Significant life changes, such as moving, getting married, having a baby, or retiring, can cause stress as people adjust to new circumstances.

7. Social stress: Social pressures, such as fitting in with a particular group, meeting new people, or public speaking, can be a source of stress for some people.

8. Environmental stress: Living in an environment with pollution, noise, or other factors that can cause discomfort or health problems can cause stress.

9. Technology-related stress: Technology-related stress can be caused by constant connectivity, social media pressure, or fear of missing out (FOMO).

10. Life transitions: Life transitions such as moving to a new home, starting a new job, or experiencing a major life change such as marriage or divorce can be stressful
These are just some of the common causes of stress in daily life. It's important to remember that everyone is different and what causes stress for one person may not cause stress for another.

Tips for improving sleep hygiene to reduce stress.

Getting enough quality sleep is crucial for overall health and well-being, both physically and mentally. Poor sleep hygiene can lead to a number of negative effects, including stress, anxiety, depression, and other health problems. In this article, we will discuss some tips for improving sleep hygiene to reduce stress.

1. Establish a regular sleep schedule: Go to bed and wake up at the same time every day, even on weekends. This helps regulate your body's internal clock, which can improve the quality of your sleep.

2. Create a relaxing sleep environment: Make your bedroom a quiet, dark, and comfortable space that is conducive to sleep. Use blackout curtains, earplugs, or a white noise machine to block out any disruptive sounds or light.

3. Limit exposure to electronic devices: Avoid using electronic devices such as smartphones, tablets, or laptops in bed. The blue light emitted by these devices can interfere with your sleep by suppressing the

production of melatonin, the hormone that regulates sleep.

4. Avoid caffeine, alcohol, and nicotine: These substances can interfere with your sleep and reduce the quality of your rest. Avoid consuming caffeine in the afternoon or evening, and limit your intake of alcohol and nicotine.

5. Exercise regularly: Regular exercise can improve the quality of your sleep, but it's important to avoid exercising too close to bedtime. Exercise can also help reduce stress and anxiety, which can improve sleep quality.

6. Practice relaxation techniques: Techniques such as deep breathing, progressive muscle relaxation, or meditation can help reduce stress and promote relaxation, which can improve sleep quality.

7. Limit daytime naps: If you must take a nap during the day, limit it to no more than 30 minutes and avoid napping late in the day.

8. Establish a bedtime routine: Develop a relaxing bedtime routine to signal to your body that it's time to sleep. This could include taking a warm bath, reading a book, or listening to soothing music.

9. Don't watch the clock: Watching the clock can increase stress and anxiety, making it harder to fall asleep. Avoid looking at the clock if you wake up during the night, and consider removing it from your bedroom altogether.

10. Consider seeking professional help: If you continue to have trouble sleeping despite making changes to your sleep hygiene, consider seeking professional help. A healthcare provider can help identify

underlying causes of sleep problems and recommend treatment options.

Improving sleep hygiene is an effective way to reduce stress and improve overall health and well-being. By establishing a regular sleep schedule, creating a relaxing sleep environment, limiting exposure to electronic devices, avoiding caffeine and alcohol, exercising regularly, practicing relaxation techniques, limiting daytime naps, establishing a bedtime routine, not watching the clock, and seeking professional help if necessary, you can improve the quality of your sleep and reduce stress in your life.

Chapter 3

The effects of chronic stress on physical and mental health.

Chronic stress is a type of stress that persists over an extended period, and it can have a profound impact on both physical and mental health. Stress is a natural response of the body to external or internal challenges, and in small doses, it can be beneficial as it can motivate us and help us deal with challenges. However, when stress becomes chronic, it can lead to serious health problems.

Physical Effects of Chronic Stress:
Chronic stress can take a significant toll on physical health. It can lead to the activation of the body's stress response system, which results in the release of stress hormones such as cortisol and adrenaline. The prolonged release of these hormones can lead to various physical symptoms, including:

1. Cardiovascular Issues: Chronic stress can cause heart disease and hypertension as the stress hormones constrict blood vessels, making it harder for the heart to pump blood.

2. Digestive Problems: Chronic stress can lead to digestive problems such as stomach ulcers, irritable bowel syndrome, and acid reflux.

3. Weakened Immune System: Chronic stress can weaken the immune system, making individuals more susceptible to infections and illnesses.

4. Chronic Pain: Chronic stress can cause or exacerbate chronic pain conditions such as headaches, back pain, and muscle tension.

5. Insomnia: Chronic stress can interfere with sleep, leading to insomnia, which can further exacerbate physical symptoms.

Mental Effects of Chronic Stress:
Chronic stress can also have a profound impact on mental health. It can lead to the development of various mental health problems, including:

1. Anxiety: Chronic stress can cause persistent feelings of worry and anxiety, making it challenging to manage daily tasks and activities.

2. Depression: Chronic stress can lead to the development of depression, which can cause feelings of sadness, hopelessness, and helplessness.

3. Cognitive Issues: Chronic stress can cause cognitive issues such as poor concentration, forgetfulness, and difficulty making decisions.

4. Substance Abuse: Chronic stress can lead to substance abuse, as individuals may turn to drugs or alcohol to cope with stress.

5. Social Withdrawal: Chronic stress can cause individuals to withdraw from social activities and relationships, leading to loneliness and isolation.
Chronic stress can have severe physical and mental health effects. It is crucial to identify and manage chronic stress to prevent the development of these health problems. Managing chronic stress involves adopting healthy lifestyle habits such as exercising, eating a healthy diet, getting enough sleep, and practicing relaxation techniques such as meditation and yoga. Seeking support from a mental health professional can also be beneficial in managing chronic stress.

Identifying your personal stress triggers and warning signs.
Stress is an unavoidable part of life, but identifying your personal stress triggers and

warning signs can help you manage and cope with stress more effectively. By recognizing what causes stress in your life and how it manifests, you can take proactive steps to reduce your stress levels and prevent it from becoming overwhelming.

Identifying Personal Stress Triggers:
Personal stress triggers are things that cause you to feel stressed. They can be different for each person, and what causes stress for one person may not necessarily cause stress for another. Some common personal stress triggers include:

1. Work-related stress: This can include job demands, a heavy workload, tight deadlines, and conflict with colleagues.

2. Relationship issues: This can include conflicts with a spouse or partner, family problems, or social isolation.

3. Financial stress: This can include financial worries, debt, and job loss.

4. Health-related stress: This can include chronic health conditions, illness, and injury.

5. Environmental stress: This can include noise, pollution, and other environmental factors that can cause stress.

Identifying Personal Stress Warning Signs: Personal stress warning signs are the physical, emotional, and behavioral cues that signal that you are experiencing stress. Some common personal stress warning signs include:

1. Physical Symptoms: These can include headaches, muscle tension, fatigue, difficulty sleeping, and gastrointestinal problems.

2. Emotional Symptoms: These can include irritability, anxiety, depression, and feeling overwhelmed.

3. Behavioral Symptoms: These can include changes in eating habits, increased use of alcohol or drugs, social withdrawal, and decreased productivity.

How to Identify Personal Stress Triggers and Warning Signs:

There are several ways to identify your personal stress triggers and warning signs, including:

1. Keeping a Stress Journal: Writing down what causes stress and how you respond to it can help you identify your personal stress triggers and warning signs.

2. Reflecting on Your Emotions: Paying attention to how you feel and what causes those feelings can help you identify personal stress triggers and warning signs.

3. Seeking Feedback: Asking friends, family members, or a mental health professional for feedback can help you identify patterns and triggers that you may not be aware of.

4. Taking a Self-Assessment: Many online self-assessment tools are available that can help you identify your personal stress triggers and warning signs.

Identifying your personal stress triggers and warning signs is an essential step in managing stress effectively. By recognizing what causes stress and how it manifests, you can take proactive steps to reduce your stress levels and prevent it from becoming overwhelming. By practicing stress management techniques and seeking support when needed, you can improve your ability to cope with stress and improve your overall well-being.

Chapter 4

How to build a support system and seek help when needed.

Having a strong support system can be essential for mental and emotional well-being. However, building a support system and seeking help when needed can be challenging for some people. In this article, we will explore some tips on how to build a support system and seek help when needed.

1. Identify your support system

The first step in building a support system is to identify the people in your life who are supportive and trustworthy. This may include family members, friends, co-workers, or mental health professionals. Make a list of people you feel comfortable talking to and who have shown they can be supportive in the past.

2. Communicate your needs

Once you have identified your support system, it is important to communicate your needs clearly. Let your loved ones know how they can best support you and what you need from them. This can include things like listening, offering advice, or just being present.

3. Cultivate positive relationships

Building a support system is not just about having people in your life, but also about cultivating positive relationships with them. Make an effort to spend time with your loved ones and engage in activities that bring you joy. This can help strengthen your relationships and make it easier to ask for help when you need it.

4. Seek professional help

Sometimes, building a support system may not be enough, and professional help may be necessary. If you are struggling with mental health issues, consider seeking the help of a mental health professional. They can provide you with the tools and support you need to manage your symptoms and improve your overall well-being.

5. Practice self-care

In addition to building a support system, it is also important to practice self-care. This can include things like getting enough sleep, eating a healthy diet, and engaging in regular exercise. Taking care of your physical health can help improve your mental and emotional well-being, making it easier to manage stress and seek help when needed.

6. Don't be afraid to ask for help

Finally, it is important to remember that asking for help is not a sign of weakness. If you are struggling, don't be afraid to reach out to your support system or a mental health professional for help. Remember, seeking help is a sign of strength, and it can help you on the path to recovery.

Building a support system and seeking help when needed can be essential for mental and emotional well-being. By identifying your support system, communicating your needs, cultivating positive relationships, seeking professional help, practicing self-care, and not being afraid to ask for help, you can build a strong support system that can help you navigate life's challenges.

Techniques for managing stress, including mindfulness, meditation, exercises

Stress is an inevitable part of our lives, but excessive stress can have adverse effects on our mental and physical health. Therefore, managing stress is crucial for maintaining a healthy and happy life. Here are some techniques for managing stress, including mindfulness and meditation:

1. Mindfulness:

Mindfulness is a technique that involves being present in the moment and being aware of your thoughts and emotions. It helps you observe your thoughts and feelings without judgment and respond to them in a more constructive way. Mindfulness techniques include:

- Breathing exercises: Mindful breathing is a simple yet effective way to reduce stress. Sit comfortably, close your eyes, and focus on your breath as you inhale and exhale. Count to four as you inhale and exhale for the same duration. If your mind wanders, gently bring your attention back to your breath.

- Body scan: This technique involves bringing your attention to each part of your body, from your toes to the top of your head. As you focus on each body part, try to release any tension or discomfort you may be experiencing.

- Mindful walking: Take a break from your daily routine and go for a walk. Focus on the sensations of your body as you walk, the movement of your feet, and the sounds around you. Try to clear your mind and focus on the present moment.

2. Meditation:

Meditation is a technique that involves training your mind to focus and relax. It helps you develop a more positive outlook on life and reduces stress and anxiety. Meditation techniques include:

- Transcendental Meditation: This technique involves sitting comfortably with your eyes closed and repeating a mantra in your mind. The mantra can be any word or phrase that has a calming effect on you.

- Loving-kindness meditation: This technique involves sending positive thoughts and feelings to yourself and others. Sit comfortably with your eyes closed and focus on sending positive energy to yourself, then to someone you love, then to someone you don't know well, and finally to someone you have a difficult relationship with.

- Body scan meditation: This technique is similar to the mindfulness body scan. Sit comfortably with your eyes closed and bring your attention to each part of your body. Release any tension or discomfort you may be experiencing.

3. Exercise:

Regular exercise is one of the most effective ways to manage stress. Exercise releases endorphins, which are natural mood-boosters. It also helps reduce muscle tension and improves sleep, which can reduce stress. Some effective exercises for stress management include:

- Yoga: Yoga involves gentle stretching and breathing exercises that help calm the mind and reduce stress. It also helps improve flexibility and balance.

- Tai Chi: Tai Chi is a low-impact exercise that involves slow, controlled movements. It helps reduce stress, improve balance, and increase flexibility.

- Aerobic exercise: Aerobic exercise, such as running, cycling, or swimming, can help reduce stress by releasing endorphins and improving overall health.

In conclusion, managing stress is essential for maintaining a healthy and happy life. Mindfulness, meditation, and exercise are effective techniques for managing stress. By incorporating these techniques into your daily routine, you can reduce stress and improve your overall well-being.

Chapter 5

Nutrition and diet tips to manage stress.

Stress can take a toll on our mental and physical health. When we are stressed, we tend to crave unhealthy foods that can worsen our stress levels. Therefore, managing stress through a healthy diet is crucial. Here are some nutrition and diet tips to manage stress:

1. Eat a balanced diet:

A balanced diet that includes a variety of fruits, vegetables, whole grains, lean proteins, and healthy fats can help reduce stress levels. A diet rich in nutrients can help maintain a healthy immune system, which is important for managing stress.

2. Reduce caffeine and sugar intake:

Caffeine and sugar can increase stress levels and cause fluctuations in energy levels. It's best to reduce or eliminate caffeine and sugar intake as much as possible.

3. Eat foods that boost serotonin:

Serotonin is a neurotransmitter that helps regulate mood, and low levels of serotonin are associated with depression and anxiety. Foods that can help boost serotonin levels include:

- Complex carbohydrates such as whole-grain bread, pasta, and brown rice
- Foods rich in omega-3 fatty acids, such as salmon, walnuts, and flaxseeds
- Foods high in tryptophan, such as turkey, chicken, eggs, and tofu

4. Include foods rich in magnesium:

Magnesium is a mineral that can help reduce stress and anxiety. Foods that are high in magnesium include:

- Leafy greens such as spinach and kale
- Nuts and seeds such as almonds, cashews, and pumpkin seeds
- Legumes such as black beans and lentils
- Whole grains such as brown rice and quinoa

5. Avoid processed foods:

Processed foods, including fast food, snacks, and desserts, are often high in sugar, unhealthy fats, and sodium. These foods can increase stress levels and cause inflammation in the body. It's best to avoid processed foods and choose whole, unprocessed foods instead.

6. Stay hydrated:

Dehydration can cause fatigue, headaches, and worsen stress levels. It's important to drink plenty of water throughout the day to stay hydrated.

7. Plan and prepare meals:

Planning and preparing meals in advance can help reduce stress and ensure that you are eating a healthy, balanced diet. Set aside time each week to plan and prepare meals, and make sure to include plenty of fruits, vegetables, lean proteins, and whole grains.

In conclusion, a healthy diet is essential for managing stress levels. Incorporating nutrient-rich foods and avoiding processed foods, caffeine, and sugar can help reduce stress and anxiety. Staying hydrated and planning and preparing meals in advance can also help maintain a healthy diet and reduce stress.

The benefits of regular self-care and relaxation practices.

Regular self-care and relaxation practices are essential for maintaining our physical and mental health. In today's fast-paced world, we often forget to take time for ourselves and prioritize self-care. However, taking care of ourselves is crucial for reducing stress, increasing our resilience, and improving our overall well-being. Here are some benefits of regular self-care and relaxation practices:

1. Reduces stress:

Stress is a common problem in today's society, and it can lead to a range of health problems, including anxiety, depression, and high blood pressure. Regular self-care and relaxation practices can help reduce stress levels by calming the nervous system, promoting relaxation, and reducing cortisol levels.

2. Improves physical health:

Self-care practices such as exercise, healthy eating, and getting enough sleep can help improve physical health. Regular exercise can help reduce the risk of chronic diseases such as heart disease, diabetes, and obesity. Eating a healthy diet can help reduce the risk of chronic diseases and improve energy levels, while getting enough sleep is essential for overall health and well-being.

3. Enhances mental health:

Self-care practices such as mindfulness, meditation, and therapy can help enhance mental health. Mindfulness and meditation can help reduce anxiety and depression, improve focus and concentration, and increase feelings of calm and relaxation. Therapy can help individuals work through emotional issues and develop coping strategies to deal with stress and anxiety.

4. Boosts self-esteem:

Self-care practices can help boost self-esteem and confidence. When we take care of ourselves, we feel better physically and mentally, which can increase our self-worth and self-esteem. Self-care practices such as getting a massage, taking a relaxing bath, or treating ourselves to something special can help improve our mood and boost our self-confidence.

5. Increases resilience:

Self-care and relaxation practices can help increase resilience and improve our ability to cope with stress and adversity. Regular exercise, meditation, and therapy can help us develop coping strategies and build a sense of inner strength and resilience that can help us navigate life's challenges.

In conclusion, regular self-care and relaxation practices are essential for maintaining our physical and mental health. By reducing stress, improving physical health, enhancing mental health, boosting self-esteem, and increasing resilience, self-care practices can help us lead happier, healthier, and more fulfilling lives. It's important to prioritize self-care and relaxation in our daily lives to ensure that we are taking care of ourselves and living our best lives.

9 798393 838720